GALVESTON DIET COOKBOOK 2024

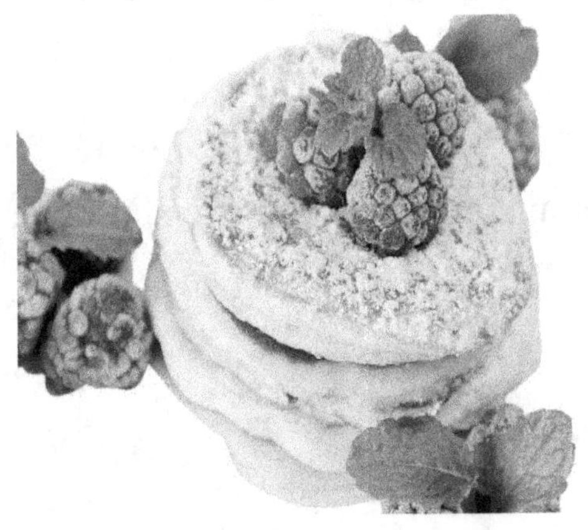

DELICIOUS RECIPES FOR A HEALTHIER YOU!

Misty J. Font

TABLE OF CONTENT

GALVESTON DIET COOKBOOK 2024..................1

CHAPTER 1: INTRODUCTION..........................7

   ABOUT THE BOOK..................................11

   ABOUT THE GALVESTON DIET..................12

CHAPTER 2: PLANNING AND PREPARATION...15

   LOOKING FOR FOOD TIPS FOR THE
GALVESTON DIET....................................16

CHAPTER 3: BREAKFAST DELIGHT.................19

   Berry Blast Smoothie Bowl.......................19

   Veggie-loaded Omelette Wraps.................20

   Almond Joy Overnight Oats.......................21

   Spinach and Feta Breakfast Quiche..............22

   Chia Seed Pudding Parfait.........................23

   Sweet Potato and Turkey Sausage Breakfast
Hash..24

   Quinoa Breakfast Bowl............................25

   Avocado and Smoked Salmon Toast.............26

   Blueberry Almond Flour Pancakes.................26

   Coconut Mango Smoothie..........................27

   Turkey and Vegetable Breakfast Burrito Bowl.28

   Apple Cinnamon Overnight Oats...................29

   Mediterranean Egg Muffins.........................30

   Banana Walnut Breakfast Cookies.................31

   Veggie and Goat Cheese Frittata...................31

CHAPTER 4: LUNCHTIME FAVORITES............33

   Quinoa Salad with Lemon-Tahini Dressing.....33

   Grilled Chicken and Vegetable Wrap.............34

   Lentil and Vegetable Stew.........................35

Mediterranean Chickpea Salad......................36

Shrimp and Avocado Salad............................37

Quinoa and Black Bean Stuffed Peppers.......38

Turkey and Vegetable Stir-Fry...................... 40

Caprese Salad with Balsamic Glaze.............. 41

Tuna and White Bean Salad.......................... 41

Sweet Potato and Black Bean Quesadillas.....42

Mediterranean Chicken Wrap......................... 44

Eggplant and Tomato Stacks......................... 44

Broccoli and Cheddar Quiche........................ 46

Asian-Inspired Salmon Salad......................... 47

Blackened Shrimp and Quinoa Bowl.............. 47

CHAPTER 5: NOURISHING DINNER.................49

Lemon Garlic Roasted Chicken...................... 49

Baked Salmon with Dill Yogurt Sauce.............50

Vegetable Stir-Fry with Tofu.......................... 51

Stuffed Bell Peppers with Turkey and Quinoa 52

Zucchini Noodles with Pesto and Cherry
Tomatoes..53

Teriyaki Chicken Stir-Fry............................... 54

Spaghetti Squash with Turkey Bolognese...... 56

Cauliflower Fried Rice with Shrimp................. 57

Mediterranean Stuffed Chicken Breast........... 59

Pesto Zoodle Bowl with Grilled Chicken......... 60

Lentil and Vegetable Curry............................. 61

Baked Eggplant Parmesan............................. 63

Black Bean and Quinoa Stuffed Peppers........64

Avocado slices for garnish............................. 65

Shrimp and Asparagus Stir-Fry......................65

Stuffed Acorn Squash with Quinoa and Kale..67

CHAPTER 6: SNACKS.................... 69

Guacamole Stuffed Cucumber Cups.............. 69

Greek Yogurt and Berry Parfait....................... 70

Spicy Roasted Chickpeas........................... 71

Caprese Skewers...................................72

Apple Slices with Almond Butter.................... 73

Hummus and Veggie Platter........................ 74

Smoked Salmon and Cucumber Bites............ 74

Berry Smoothie Bowl................................75

Edamame and Sea Salt Pods......................... 76

Baked Sweet Potato Chips........................... 76

Avocado and Tomato Salsa....................... 77

Nut and Seed Trail Mix..............................79

Cottage Cheese with Pineapple Chunks........ 80

Stuffed Bell Pepper Halves........................... 80

Rice Cake with Almond Butter and Banana Slices..81

CHAPTER 7: DESSERTS AND TREATS............ 83

Chocolate Avocado Mousse........................... 83

Almond Flour Blueberry Muffins..................... 84

Chia Seed Chocolate Pudding....................... 85

Coconut Flour Banana Bread...................... 86

Berry and Almond Flour Crisp........................88

Avocado Chocolate Chip Cookies.................. 89

Greek Yogurt Parfait with Honey and Berries. 90

Pumpkin Spice Chia Pudding........................ 91

Almond Butter Energy Bites........................... 92

Coconut Lime Energy Balls............................93

Chocolate Covered Strawberries.................... 94

Cinnamon Baked Apples.............................95

Mixed Berry Sorbet............................ 96

Lemon Poppy Seed Muffins........................ 97

Raspberry Coconut Chia Popsicles............... 98

CHAPTER 8: SMOOTHIE AND BEVERAGES RECIPES... 101

Green Detox Smoothie.............................101

Berry Protein Smoothie........................ 102

Tropical Turmeric Smoothie........................ 103

Cucumber Mint Cooler................................ 104

Golden Milk Latte.................................... 105

Blueberry Avocado Smoothie........................106

Minty Watermelon Refresher........................ 107

Chocolate Peanut Butter Protein Shake....... 108

Pineapple Ginger Turmeric Elixir................. 109

Vanilla Almond Chai Smoothie..................... 110

Raspberry Coconut Water Refresher........... 111

Matcha Green Tea Latte.............................112

Orange Creamsicle Smoothie...................... 113

Peach Mint Iced Tea................................114

Coconut Berry Smoothie Bowl..................... 115

CONCLUSION..117

ADDITIONAL RESOURCES........................ 117

CHAPTER 1: INTRODUCTION

the delightful ocean front town of Galveston, Paul's life wandered off in a peculiar course when prosperity challenges represented a likely danger over his once-dynamic presence. Fighting with the repercussions of an unbalanced lifestyle, he ended up at a convergence, yearning for a response that wouldn't simply address his prosperity concerns yet moreover give a pragmatic way to recovery. Much to his consternation that his salvation would come as the Galveston Diet Cookbook, a culinary helper that would transform into the underpinning of his interaction back to criticalness.

Paul's prosperity fights were different, consolidating issues like weight the board, exhaustion, and a general sensation of distress. Regular eating regimens had bombarded him, leaving him incapacitated and skeptical about the chance of finding a philosophy that could truly make a difference. That was until he unintentionally found the Galveston Diet Cookbook, a thorough rundown of recipes unequivocally planned to help in everyday prosperity and success.

As Paul dove into the pages of the cookbook, he tracked down some different option from a variety of recipes; he tracked down a manual for far reaching prosperity. The Galveston Diet, delineated in the cookbook, focused on the significance of supporting the body with whole, supplement thick food sources while keeping a fair method for managing sustenance. It wasn't just an eating schedule; it was a lifestyle that resounded with Paul's hankering for a legitimate and noteworthy change.

The cookbook offered an alternate display of recipes, going from enticing principal courses to empowering rewards and perfect desserts. Each recipe was made with an exacting perception of healthy guidelines, ensuring that Paul participated in his suppers as well as outfitted his body with the major construction blocks for recovery. The emphasis on uniting quieting food sources and zeroing in on a sensible extent of macronutrients transformed into the guiding principle that Paul expected to recuperate control over his prosperity.

Paul's culinary trip was an examination of flavors, surfaces, and the retouching properties of food. Whether savoring a unique Mediterranean plate of leafy greens rich in cell fortifications or partaking in a satisfyingly solid sweet potato and dull bean bowl, each dish transformed into an exhibit of the uncommon impact of purposeful, prosperity focused eating.

Past the genuine perspectives, the Galveston Diet Cookbook granted in Paul a re-energized sensation of care about his relationship with food. It wasn't just about calories and parts; it was connected to empowering a positive and reasonable relationship with the food his body justified. The cookbook transformed into Paul's accepted companion, guiding him through the intricacies of dining experience orchestrating, looking for food, and, shockingly, culinary experimentation.

As weeks changed into months, Paul's prosperity began to give signs of a striking circle back. The weight he stressed over as a worry lifted, displaced by a newfound power and importance. The weariness that had once harassed every one of his means gave way to deal with upheld energy levels. The Galveston Diet Cookbook turned into a combination of recipes as well as an account of Paul's solidarity, confirmation, and outrageous triumph over prosperity challenges.

Paul's story is a show of the phenomenal potential embedded in the Galveston Diet Cookbook. It is an account of recovery, fortifying, and the tremendous impact that intentional and supporting food choices can have on one's interaction back to prosperity. Through the pages of the cookbook, Paul found the recipes for recovery as well as the keys to opening a superior, more unique life in the coastline safe house of

ABOUT THE BOOK

Welcome to the Galveston Diet Cookbook, a culinary buddy created to improve and raise your excursion towards a better and more dynamic way of life. Established in the standards of the Galveston Diet, this cookbook is intended to give heavenly and fulfilling recipes as well as to offer a thorough aide on embracing a practical and supporting approach to eating.

ABOUT THE GALVESTON DIET

The Galveston Diet is something other than a dietary arrangement; a comprehensive way to deal with wellbeing underlines the extraordinary wholesome requirements of ladies, considering hormonal vacillations and advancing equilibrium from the inside. Dr. Mary Claire Haver, the visionary behind the Galveston Diet, has enabled incalculable people to recover their wellbeing and essentialness through this proof based approach.

The Philosophy Behind the Cookbook

This cookbook isn't simply an assortment of recipes; it's a sign of the Galveston Diet reasoning. Each dish is insightfully made to focus on supplement thickness, flavor, and effortlessness, making it open to both prepared home cooks and those moving into the kitchen. We want to demonstrate the way that good dieting can be a cheerful and tasty experience.

Getting Started with the Galveston Diet

Whether you're a novice to the Galveston Diet or a carefully prepared professional, this segment gives an establishment to progress. We'll investigate the center standards of the Galveston Diet, demystify normal misguided judgments, and guide you through the underlying strides of carrying out this extraordinary way to deal with eating.

Set out on this culinary experience with us, where sustaining your body turns into a festival of flavors, and each dinner is a valuable chance to respect your prosperity. The Galveston Diet Cookbook is in excess of a recipe assortment; it's a sidekick on your excursion to wellbeing, essentialness, and a recharged association with the food you eat.

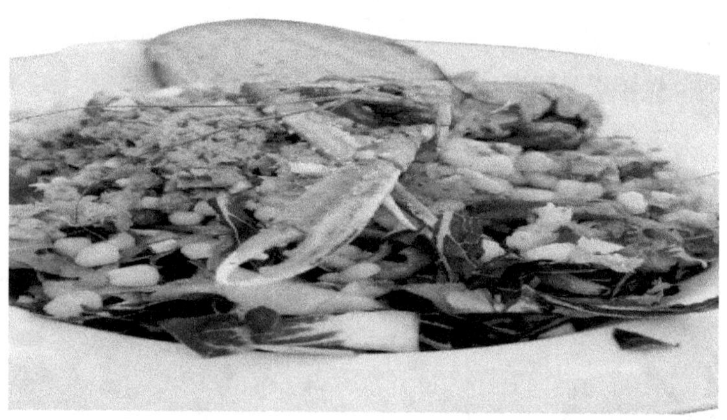

CHAPTER 2: PLANNING AND PREPARATION

Effective and careful feast arranging is a foundation of progress on the Galveston Diet. In this section, we guide you through the most common way of making balanced, fulfilling dinners that line up with the standards of the Galveston Diet.

Building a Balanced Plate

Find the craft of developing a Galveston Diet-accommodating plate that ideally upholds hormonal equilibrium and generally speaking prosperity. We investigate segment control, the significance of consolidating various supplement thick food sources, and the job of macronutrients in making dinners that stimulate and support.

Weekly Meal Planning Guide

Explore the week ahead with our thorough dinner arranging guide. From breakfast to supper and in the middle between, we give commonsense tips to organizing your feasts over time. Figure out how to integrate different flavors, surfaces, and nourishing parts into your week after week menu, guaranteeing a delightful and changed diet.

LOOKING FOR FOOD TIPS FOR THE GALVESTON DIET

Make your looking for food experience a breeze with our coordinated summary of Galveston Diet-embraced trimmings. We offer encounters into picking the freshest produce, picking lean proteins, and recognizing sound fats, drawing in you to go with informed choices at the corner store.

Explore productive systems and sort out some way to stock your kitchen with nuts and bolts that line up with the Galveston Diet.

Proficient Supper Prep Philosophies

Viability meets food with our productive gala prep frameworks. Track down how to design parts of your meals somewhat early, ensuring that you have nutritious and sublime options speedily available. We give tips on bunch cooking, limit techniques, and creating adaptable parts that can be reused over the long haul.

Area 2 outfits you with the helpful instruments expected to immaculately integrate the Galveston Diet into your everyday daily practice. From orchestrating your blowouts to investigating the general store with assurance, you'll be all set to leave on a journey of reviving and satisfying eating.

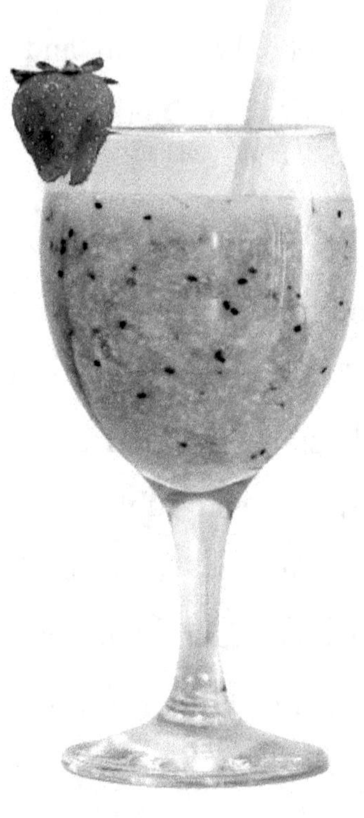

CHAPTER 3: BREAKFAST DELIGHT

Berry Blast Smoothie Bowl

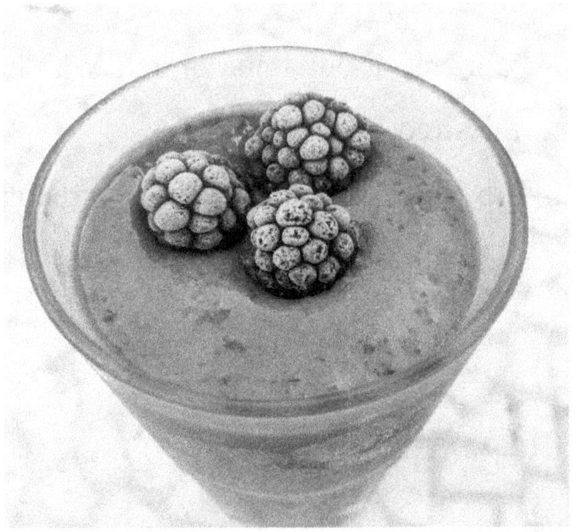

Ingredients:

- 1 cup mixed berries (strawberries, blueberries, raspberries)
- 1 banana, frozen
- 1/2 cup Greek yogurt
- 1 tablespoon chia seeds
- 1/2 cup almond milk

- 1 tablespoon honey (optional)

Instructions:

1. Blend berries, frozen banana, Greek yogurt, chia seeds, and almond milk until smooth.
2. Pour into a bowl and drizzle with honey if desired.
3. Top with additional berries, granola, or sliced almonds for added texture.

Veggie-loaded Omelette Wraps

Ingredients:

- 4 eggs, beaten
- 1/2 cup spinach, chopped
- 1/4 cup cherry tomatoes, diced
- 1/4 cup bell peppers, diced
- 1/4 cup feta cheese, crumbled
- Salt and pepper to taste

- 2 whole wheat tortillas

Instructions:

1. In a bowl, mix together beaten eggs, spinach, tomatoes, bell peppers, and feta cheese.
2. Season with salt and pepper.
3. Pour the mixture into a heated non-stick skillet and cook until the eggs are set.
4. Spoon the omelette onto whole wheat tortillas, roll, and serve.

Almond Joy Overnight Oats

Ingredients:

- 1/2 cup old-fashioned oats
- 1/2 cup almond milk
- 1 tablespoon almond butter
- 1 tablespoon shredded coconut
- 1 tablespoon dark chocolate chips

- 1/2 banana, sliced

Instructions:

1. In a jar, combine oats, almond milk, almond butter, shredded coconut, and dark chocolate chips.
2. Stir well, cover, and refrigerate overnight.
3. In the morning, top with sliced banana before serving.

Spinach and Feta Breakfast Quiche

Ingredients:

- 4 eggs, beaten
- 1 cup spinach, chopped
- 1/4 cup feta cheese, crumbled
- 1/4 cup red onion, diced
- Salt and pepper to taste

Instructions:

1. Preheat the oven to 350°F (175°C).

2. In a bowl, combine beaten eggs, spinach, feta cheese, red onion, salt, and pepper.

3. Pour the mixture into a greased pie dish and bake for 25-30 minutes or until the quiche is set.

Chia Seed Pudding Parfait

Ingredients:

1. 2 tablespoons chia seeds
2. 1/2 cup almond milk
3. 1/2 teaspoon vanilla extract
4. 1/4 cup granola
5. 1/2 cup mixed berries

Instructions:

1. In a jar, mix chia seeds, almond milk, and vanilla extract.

2. Stir well, cover, and refrigerate for at least 2 hours or overnight.

3. Layer the chia seed pudding with granola and mixed berries in a glass.

Sweet Potato and Turkey Sausage Breakfast Hash

Ingredients:

- 1 sweet potato, diced
- 1/2 pound turkey sausage, crumbled
- 1 bell pepper, diced
- 1/2 red onion, diced
- 2 tablespoons olive oil
- Salt and pepper to taste

Instructions:

1. In a skillet, heat olive oil over medium heat.

2. Add sweet potato, turkey sausage, bell pepper, and red onion.

3. Cook until the sweet potato is tender and the sausage is cooked through.

4. Season with salt and pepper and serve.

Quinoa Breakfast Bowl

Ingredients:

- 1 cup cooked quinoa
- 1/2 cup almond milk
- 1 tablespoon honey
- 1/4 cup sliced almonds
- 1/2 cup mixed fruit (berries, banana)

Instructions:

1. In a bowl, combine cooked quinoa, almond milk, honey, and sliced almonds.

2. Top with mixed fruit before serving.

Avocado and Smoked Salmon Toast

Ingredients:

- 2 slices whole grain bread, toasted
- 1/2 avocado, mashed
- 4 ounces smoked salmon
- 1 tablespoon capers
- Fresh dill for garnish

Instructions:

1. Spread mashed avocado on toasted bread slices.
2. Top with smoked salmon, capers, and fresh dill.

Blueberry Almond Flour Pancakes

Ingredients:

- 1 cup almond flour
- 2 eggs
- 1/2 cup almond milk

- 1 teaspoon baking powder
- 1/2 cup blueberries

Instructions:

1. In a bowl, whisk together almond flour, eggs, almond milk, and baking powder.
2. Gently fold in blueberries.
3. Cook pancakes on a griddle over medium heat until golden brown.

Coconut Mango Smoothie

Ingredients:

- 1 cup mango chunks, frozen
- 1/2 cup coconut milk
- 1/2 cup Greek yogurt
- 1 tablespoon shredded coconut

Instructions:

1. Blend mango chunks, coconut milk, and Greek yogurt until smooth.

2. Pour into a glass and sprinkle with shredded coconut.

Turkey and Vegetable Breakfast Burrito Bowl

Ingredients:

- 1/2 cup cooked quinoa
- 1/2 cup black beans, drained and rinsed
- 1/2 cup ground turkey, cooked
- 1/4 cup salsa
- 1/4 cup shredded cheese
- Avocado slices for garnish

Instructions:

1. In a bowl, layer cooked quinoa, black beans, ground turkey, salsa, and shredded cheese.

2. Microwave or heat in a skillet until warmed through.

3. Garnish with avocado slices before serving.

Apple Cinnamon Overnight Oats

Ingredients:

- 1/2 cup old-fashioned oats
- 1/2 cup almond milk
- 1/2 apple, diced
- 1 tablespoon maple syrup
- 1/2 teaspoon cinnamon

Instructions:

1. In a jar, combine oats, almond milk, diced apple, maple syrup, and cinnamon.

2. Stir well, cover, and refrigerate overnight.

3. Stir again before serving.

Mediterranean Egg Muffins

Ingredients:

- 6 eggs, beaten
- 1/2 cup cherry tomatoes, halved
- 1/4 cup feta cheese, crumbled
- 2 tablespoons black olives, sliced
- 1 tablespoon fresh parsley, chopped

Instructions:

1. Preheat the oven to 375°F (190°C).
2. In a bowl, mix together beaten eggs, cherry tomatoes, feta cheese, black olives, and parsley.
3. Pour the mixture into greased muffin tins and bake for 15-18 minutes or until set.

Banana Walnut Breakfast Cookies

Ingredients:

- 2 ripe bananas, mashed
- 1 cup old-fashioned oats
- 1/4 cup chopped walnuts
- 1/4 cup raisins
- 1 teaspoon vanilla extract

Instructions:

1. Preheat the oven to 350°F (175°C).
2. In a bowl, combine mashed bananas, oats, walnuts, raisins, and vanilla extract.
3. Drop spoonfuls of the mixture onto a baking sheet and bake for 12-15 minutes or until golden.

Veggie and Goat Cheese Frittata

Ingredients:

- 8 eggs, beaten

- 1/2 cup cherry tomatoes, halved
- 1/2 cup spinach, chopped
- 1/4 cup goat cheese, crumbled
- Salt and pepper to taste

Instructions:

1. Preheat the oven to 375°F (190°C).
2. In an oven-safe skillet, sauté cherry tomatoes and spinach until wilted.
3. Pour beaten eggs over the vegetables and sprinkle with goat cheese.
4. Season with salt and pepper, then bake for 20-25 minutes or until the frittata is set.

CHAPTER 4: LUNCHTIME FAVORITES

Quinoa Salad with Lemon-Tahini Dressing

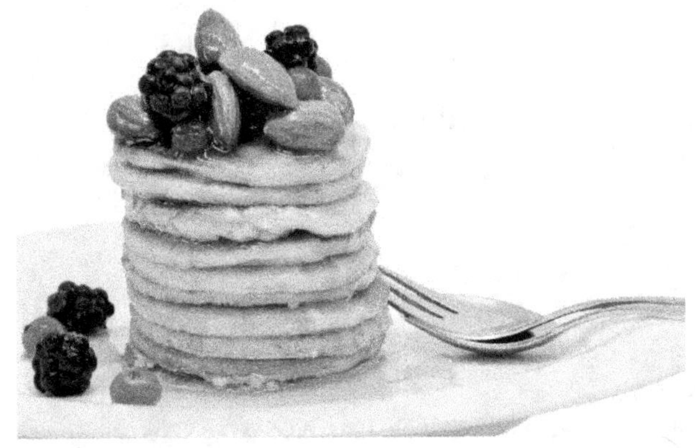

Ingredients:

- 1 cup cooked quinoa
- 1 cup cherry tomatoes, halved
- 1 cucumber, diced
- 1/4 cup red onion, finely chopped
- 1/4 cup feta cheese, crumbled
- 2 tablespoons fresh parsley, chopped

Instructions:

1. In a bowl, combine cooked quinoa, cherry tomatoes, cucumber, red onion, feta cheese, and parsley.
2. In a separate small bowl, whisk together lemon-tahini dressing.
3. Drizzle the dressing over the salad and toss to combine.

Grilled Chicken and Vegetable Wrap

Ingredients:

- 1 boneless, skinless chicken breast
- 1 whole wheat wrap
- 1/2 cup mixed bell peppers, sliced
- 1/4 cup red onion, sliced
- 1 tablespoon olive oil

- Salt and pepper to taste

Instructions:

1. Season chicken breast with salt and pepper.
2. Grill the chicken until cooked through.
3. In a skillet, sauté bell peppers and red onion in olive oil until tender.
4. Slice the grilled chicken and place it in a whole wheat wrap with sautéed vegetables.

Lentil and Vegetable Stew

Ingredients:

- 1 cup dried green lentils, rinsed
- 4 cups vegetable broth
- 1 carrot, diced
- 1 celery stalk, diced
- 1 onion, diced

- 2 cloves garlic, minced
- 1 teaspoon cumin
- 1 teaspoon smoked paprika
- Salt and pepper to taste

Instructions:

1. In a pot, combine lentils, vegetable broth, carrot, celery, onion, garlic, cumin, and smoked paprika.
2. Bring to a boil, then reduce heat and simmer until lentils are tender.
3. Season with salt and pepper before serving.

Mediterranean Chickpea Salad

Ingredients:

- 1 can (15 oz) chickpeas, drained and rinsed
- 1 cup cherry tomatoes, halved

- 1 cucumber, diced

- 1/4 cup red onion, finely chopped

- 1/4 cup Kalamata olives, sliced

- 1/4 cup feta cheese, crumbled

- 2 tablespoons fresh mint, chopped

Instructions:

- In a bowl, combine chickpeas, cherry tomatoes, cucumber, red onion, olives, feta cheese, and mint.

- Drizzle with olive oil and toss gently to combine.

Shrimp and Avocado Salad

Ingredients:

- 1/2 pound shrimp, peeled and deveined

- 1 avocado, sliced

- 1 cup mixed greens

- 1/2 cup cherry tomatoes, halved

- 2 tablespoons cilantro, chopped

- 1 tablespoon olive oil

- Juice of 1 lime

- Salt and pepper to taste

Instructions:

1. Season shrimp with salt and pepper and sauté in olive oil until cooked.

2. In a bowl, combine mixed greens, cherry tomatoes, avocado, and cooked shrimp.

3. Drizzle with lime juice and toss gently.

4. Garnish with chopped cilantro before serving.

Quinoa and Black Bean Stuffed Peppers

Ingredients:

- 4 bell peppers, halved

- 1 cup cooked quinoa

- 1 can (15 oz) black beans, drained and rinsed
- 1 cup corn kernels
- 1/2 cup salsa
- 1 teaspoon cumin
- 1/2 teaspoon chili powder
- Salt and pepper to taste

Instructions:

1. Preheat the oven to 375°F (190°C).
2. In a bowl, mix together cooked quinoa, black beans, corn, salsa, cumin, and chili powder.
3. Stuff each bell pepper half with the quinoa mixture.
4. Bake for 25-30 minutes or until peppers are tender.

Turkey and Vegetable Stir-Fry

Ingredients:

- 1/2 pound ground turkey
- 2 cups broccoli florets
- 1 bell pepper, sliced
- 1 carrot, julienned
- 2 tablespoons soy sauce
- 1 tablespoon sesame oil
- 1 tablespoon fresh ginger, grated
- 2 cloves garlic, minced

Instructions:

1. In a wok or skillet, brown ground turkey until cooked.
2. Add broccoli, bell pepper, carrot, soy sauce, sesame oil, ginger, and garlic.
3. Stir-fry until vegetables are tender-crisp.

Caprese Salad with Balsamic Glaze

Ingredients:

- 2 cups cherry tomatoes, halved
- 1 cup fresh mozzarella, diced
- 1/4 cup fresh basil leaves
- 2 tablespoons balsamic glaze
- Salt and pepper to taste

Instructions:

1. Arrange cherry tomatoes, fresh mozzarella, and basil on a serving platter.
2. Drizzle with balsamic glaze.
3. Season with salt and pepper before serving.

Tuna and White Bean Salad

Ingredients:

- 1 can (5 oz) tuna, drained

- 1 can (15 oz) white beans, drained and rinsed
- 1/2 red onion, finely chopped
- 1/4 cup fresh parsley, chopped
- 2 tablespoons olive oil
- Juice of 1 lemon
- Salt and pepper to taste

Instructions:

1. In a bowl, combine tuna, white beans, red onion, and parsley.
2. Drizzle with olive oil and lemon juice.
3. Season with salt and pepper and toss gently.

Sweet Potato and Black Bean Quesadillas

Ingredients:

- 2 whole wheat tortillas

- 1 sweet potato, cooked and mashed
- 1/2 cup black beans, mashed
- 1/2 cup spinach, chopped
- 1/4 cup shredded cheddar cheese
- 1 teaspoon cumin
- 1/2 teaspoon chili powder

Instructions:

1. In a bowl, mix together mashed sweet potato, black beans, spinach, cumin, and chili powder.
2. Spread the mixture on one side of each tortilla.
3. Sprinkle shredded cheddar cheese on top and fold in half.
4. Cook on a griddle until the tortilla is golden and the cheese is melted.

Mediterranean Chicken Wrap

Ingredients:

- 1 grilled chicken breast, sliced
- 1 whole wheat wrap
- 1/4 cup hummus
- 1/2 cup cucumber, sliced
- 1/4 cup cherry tomatoes, halved
- 2 tablespoons feta cheese, crumbled

Instructions:

- Spread hummus on a whole wheat wrap.
- Layer with sliced grilled chicken, cucumber, cherry tomatoes, and feta cheese.
- Roll up the wrap and slice in half before serving.

Eggplant and Tomato Stacks

Ingredients:

- 1 large eggplant, sliced
- 1 large tomato, sliced
- 1/4 cup fresh mozzarella, sliced
- 2 tablespoons balsamic glaze
- Fresh basil leaves for garnish
- Salt and pepper to taste

Instructions:

1. Preheat the oven to 375°F (190°C).
2. Arrange slices of eggplant and tomato on a baking sheet.
3. Top each eggplant slice with a slice of mozzarella.
4. Bake for 15-20 minutes or until the cheese is melted.
5. Drizzle with balsamic glaze, garnish with fresh basil, and season with salt and pepper.

Broccoli and Cheddar Quiche

Ingredients:

- 1 whole wheat pie crust
- 4 eggs, beaten
- 1 cup broccoli florets, steamed
- 1/2 cup sharp cheddar cheese, shredded
- 1/2 cup milk
- 1/4 teaspoon nutmeg
- Salt and pepper to taste

Instructions:

1. Preheat the oven to 375°F (190°C).
2. In a bowl, mix together beaten eggs, steamed broccoli, cheddar cheese, milk, nutmeg, salt, and pepper.
3. Pour the mixture into the whole wheat pie crust.
4. Bake for 30-35 minutes or until the quiche is set.

Asian-Inspired Salmon Salad

Ingredients:

- 1 salmon fillet, grilled
- 2 cups mixed greens
- 1/2 cup snow peas, sliced
- 1/4 cup shredded carrots
- 2 tablespoons sesame ginger dressing
- 1 tablespoon sesame seeds

Instructions:

1. Place grilled salmon on a bed of mixed greens.
2. Scatter sliced snow peas and shredded carrots on top.
3. Drizzle with sesame ginger dressing and sprinkle with sesame seeds.

Blackened Shrimp and Quinoa Bowl

Ingredients:

- 1/2 pound shrimp, blackened

- 1 cup cooked quinoa

- 1 cup mixed vegetables (bell peppers, zucchini, cherry tomatoes), grilled

- 2 tablespoons olive oil

- Juice of 1 lime

- Fresh cilantro for garnish

- Salt and pepper to taste

Instructions:

1. In a bowl, combine blackened shrimp, cooked quinoa, and grilled vegetables.

2. Drizzle with olive oil and lime juice.

3. Toss gently and garnish with fresh cilantro before serving.

CHAPTER 5: NOURISHING DINNER

Lemon Garlic Roasted Chicken

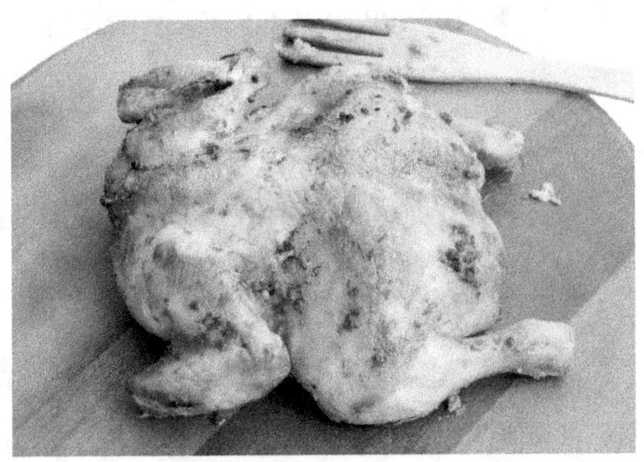

Ingredients:

- 4 boneless, skinless chicken breasts
- 2 lemons, juiced
- 4 cloves garlic, minced
- 2 tablespoons olive oil
- 1 teaspoon dried oregano
- Salt and pepper to taste

Instructions:

1. Preheat the oven to 400°F (200°C).
2. In a bowl, mix lemon juice, minced garlic, olive oil, dried oregano, salt, and pepper.
3. Place chicken breasts in a baking dish and pour the lemon-garlic mixture over them.
4. Bake for 25-30 minutes or until the chicken is cooked through.

Baked Salmon with Dill Yogurt Sauce

Ingredients:

- 4 salmon fillets
- 1/2 cup Greek yogurt
- 2 tablespoons fresh dill, chopped
- 1 tablespoon lemon juice
- 1 clove garlic, minced

- Salt and pepper to taste

Instructions:

1. Preheat the oven to 375°F (190°C).

2. Place salmon fillets on a baking sheet.

3. In a bowl, mix Greek yogurt, dill, lemon juice, minced garlic, salt, and pepper.

4. Spread the yogurt sauce over the salmon and bake for 15-20 minutes or until the salmon flakes easily.

Vegetable Stir-Fry with Tofu

Ingredients:

- 1 block extra-firm tofu, pressed and cubed
- 2 cups broccoli florets
- 1 bell pepper, sliced
- 1 carrot, julienned
- 2 tablespoons soy sauce

- 1 tablespoon hoisin sauce
- 1 tablespoon sesame oil
- 1 tablespoon fresh ginger, grated
- 2 cloves garlic, minced

Instructions:

1. In a wok or skillet, sauté tofu until golden brown.
2. Add broccoli, bell pepper, carrot, soy sauce, hoisin sauce, sesame oil, ginger, and garlic.
3. Stir-fry until vegetables are tender-crisp.

Stuffed Bell Peppers with Turkey and Quinoa

Ingredients:

- 4 bell peppers, halved
- 1/2 pound ground turkey
- 1 cup cooked quinoa

- 1 cup black beans, drained and rinsed

- 1 cup corn kernels

- 1 cup salsa

- 1 teaspoon cumin

- 1/2 teaspoon chili powder

- Salt and pepper to taste

Instructions:

1. Preheat the oven to 375°F (190°C).

2. In a bowl, mix together cooked quinoa, ground turkey, black beans, corn, salsa, cumin, and chili powder.

3. Stuff each bell pepper half with the quinoa mixture.

4. Bake for 25-30 minutes or until peppers are tender.

Zucchini Noodles with Pesto and Cherry Tomatoes

Ingredients:

- 4 medium zucchini, spiralized
- 1 cup cherry tomatoes, halved
- 1/2 cup pine nuts
- 1 cup fresh basil leaves
- 1/2 cup Parmesan cheese, grated
- 2 cloves garlic
- 1/2 cup olive oil
- Salt and pepper to taste

Instructions:

In a blender, combine pine nuts, basil, Parmesan cheese, garlic, salt, and pepper.

With the blender running, slowly add olive oil until the pesto is smooth.

Toss spiralized zucchini with pesto and cherry tomatoes.

Teriyaki Chicken Stir-Fry

Ingredients:

- 1 pound boneless, skinless chicken thighs, sliced
- 2 cups broccoli florets
- 1 bell pepper, sliced
- 1 carrot, julienned
- 1/4 cup low-sodium soy sauce
- 2 tablespoons honey
- 1 tablespoon rice vinegar
- 1 tablespoon sesame oil
- 1 tablespoon cornstarch
- 1 tablespoon water
- Sesame seeds for garnish

Instructions:

1. In a bowl, whisk together soy sauce, honey, rice vinegar, and sesame oil.
2. In a wok or skillet, sauté chicken until cooked through.

3. Add broccoli, bell pepper, and carrot.

4. Pour the teriyaki sauce over the chicken and vegetables.

5. In a small bowl, mix cornstarch and water to create a slurry.

6. Stir the slurry into the stir-fry until the sauce thickens.

7. Garnish with sesame seeds before serving.

Spaghetti Squash with Turkey Bolognese

Ingredients:

- 1 medium spaghetti squash, halved and seeds removed
- 1/2 pound ground turkey
- 1 cup tomato sauce
- 1/2 onion, finely chopped
- 2 cloves garlic, minced

- 1 teaspoon dried oregano

- 1 teaspoon dried basil

- Salt and pepper to taste

- Fresh parsley for garnish

Instructions:

1. Preheat the oven to 375°F (190°C).

2. Place spaghetti squash halves cut-side down on a baking sheet.

3. Bake for 40-45 minutes or until the squash is tender.

4. In a skillet, brown ground turkey, then add onion and garlic.

5. Stir in tomato sauce, oregano, basil, salt, and pepper.

6. Use a fork to scrape the spaghetti squash into strands.

7. Top with turkey Bolognese and garnish with fresh parsley.

Cauliflower Fried Rice with Shrimp

Ingredients:

1. 1 pound shrimp, peeled and deveined
2. 1 head cauliflower, grated
3. 1 cup mixed vegetables (peas, carrots, corn)
4. 2 eggs, beaten
5. 2 tablespoons low-sodium soy sauce
6. 1 tablespoon sesame oil
7. 1 tablespoon fresh ginger, grated
8. 2 cloves garlic, minced
9. Green onions for garnish

Instructions:

1. In a wok or skillet, sauté shrimp until cooked through.
2. Add grated cauliflower, mixed vegetables, soy sauce, sesame oil, ginger, and garlic.

3. Push the cauliflower mixture to the side
   of the pan and pour beaten eggs into the
   empty space.

4. Scramble the eggs until cooked, then mix
   them into the cauliflower mixture.

5. Garnish with green onions before
   serving.

Mediterranean Stuffed Chicken Breast

Ingredients:

- 4 boneless, skinless chicken breasts
- 1 cup cherry tomatoes, halved
- 1/2 cup Kalamata olives, sliced
- 1/4 cup feta cheese, crumbled
- 2 tablespoons fresh oregano, chopped
- 2 tablespoons olive oil
- Salt and pepper to taste

Instructions:

1. Preheat the oven to 400°F (200°C).

2. In a bowl, combine cherry tomatoes, Kalamata olives, feta cheese, fresh oregano, olive oil, salt, and pepper.

3. Cut a pocket into each chicken breast and stuff with the Mediterranean mixture.

4. Bake for 25-30 minutes or until the chicken is cooked through.

Pesto Zoodle Bowl with Grilled Chicken

Ingredients:

- 2 zucchinis, spiralized
- 1 cup cherry tomatoes, halved
- 1/2 cup artichoke hearts, chopped
- 1/4 cup pine nuts
- 1/4 cup Parmesan cheese, grated

- 1/2 cup fresh basil leaves

- 2 tablespoons olive oil

- 1 tablespoon lemon juice

- 1 clove garlic

- 4 grilled chicken breasts

Instructions:

1. In a blender, combine pine nuts, Parmesan cheese, fresh basil, olive oil, lemon juice, and garlic.

2. Spiralize zucchinis and toss with cherry tomatoes and artichoke hearts.

3. Drizzle pesto over the zoodle mixture and toss to combine.

4. Serve grilled chicken on top of the pesto zoodles.

Lentil and Vegetable Curry

Ingredients:

- 1 cup dried green lentils, rinsed
- 4 cups vegetable broth
- 1 onion, finely chopped
- 2 cloves garlic, minced
- 1 tablespoon curry powder
- 1 teaspoon ground turmeric
- 1 can (14 oz) diced tomatoes
- 1 can (14 oz) coconut milk
- 2 cups mixed vegetables (carrots, peas, bell peppers)
- Salt and pepper to taste

Instructions:

1. In a pot, combine lentils, vegetable broth, onion, garlic, curry powder, turmeric, diced tomatoes, and coconut milk.
2. Bring to a boil, then reduce heat and simmer until lentils are tender.
3. Add mixed vegetables and simmer until vegetables are cooked.

4. Season with salt and pepper before
   serving.

Baked Eggplant Parmesan

Ingredients:

- 1 large eggplant, sliced
- 1 cup whole wheat breadcrumbs
- 1/2 cup Parmesan cheese, grated
- 2 eggs, beaten
- 2 cups marinara sauce
- 1 cup mozzarella cheese, shredded
- Fresh basil for garnish
- Salt and pepper to taste

Instructions:

1. Preheat the oven to 375°F (190°C).
2. Dip eggplant slices in beaten eggs, then
   coat with a mixture of breadcrumbs,
   Parmesan cheese, salt, and pepper.

3. Arrange the coated eggplant slices in a baking dish.

4. Bake for 20-25 minutes or until the eggplant is golden.

5. In a separate bowl, mix marinara sauce with mozzarella cheese.

6. Pour the sauce over the baked eggplant and bake for an additional 15 minutes.

7. Garnish with fresh basil before serving.

Black Bean and Quinoa Stuffed Peppers

Ingredients:

- 4 bell peppers, halved
- 1 cup cooked quinoa
- 1 can (15 oz) black beans, drained and rinsed
- 1 cup corn kernels
- 1/2 cup salsa

- 1 teaspoon cumin

- 1/2 teaspoon chili powder

- Salt and pepper to taste

Avocado slices for garnish

Instructions:

1. Preheat the oven to 375°F (190°C).

2. In a bowl, mix together cooked quinoa, black beans, corn, salsa, cumin, and chili powder.

3. Stuff each bell pepper half with the quinoa mixture.

4. Bake for 25-30 minutes or until peppers are tender.

5. Garnish with avocado slices before serving.

Shrimp and Asparagus Stir-Fry

Ingredients:

- 1 pound shrimp, peeled and deveined
- 1 bunch asparagus, trimmed and cut into bite-sized pieces
- 1 red bell pepper, sliced
- 2 tablespoons low-sodium soy sauce
- 1 tablespoon hoisin sauce
- 1 tablespoon sesame oil
- 1 tablespoon fresh ginger, grated
- 2 cloves garlic, minced

Instructions:

1. In a wok or skillet, sauté shrimp until cooked through.
2. Add asparagus, red bell pepper, soy sauce, hoisin sauce, sesame oil, ginger, and garlic.
3. Stir-fry until vegetables are tender-crisp.

Stuffed Acorn Squash with Quinoa and Kale

Ingredients:

- 2 acorn squash, halved and seeds removed
- 1 cup cooked quinoa
- 1 cup kale, chopped
- 1/4 cup dried cranberries
- 1/4 cup pecans, chopped
- 2 tablespoons olive oil
- 1 tablespoon balsamic vinegar
- Salt and pepper to taste

Instructions:

1. Preheat the oven to 400°F (200°C).
2. Place acorn squash halves cut-side down on a baking sheet and bake for 30 minutes.
3. In a bowl, combine cooked quinoa, chopped kale, dried cranberries, pecans,

olive oil, balsamic vinegar, salt, and pepper.

4. Spoon the quinoa mixture into the roasted acorn squash halves.

5. Bake for an additional 15

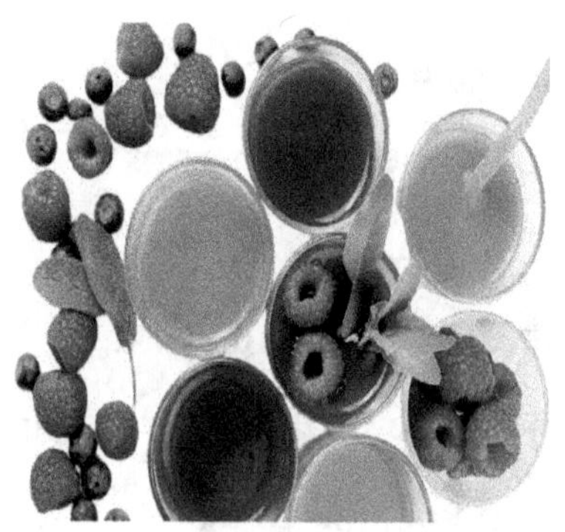

CHAPTER 6: SNACKS

Guacamole Stuffed Cucumber Cups

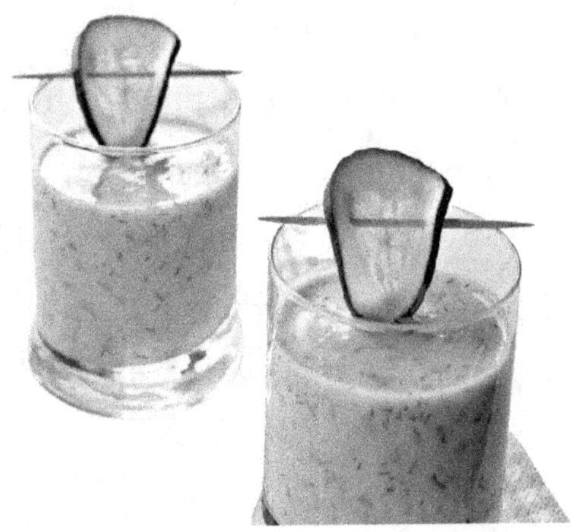

Ingredients:

- 2 large cucumbers, sliced into rounds
- 2 ripe avocados, mashed
- 1/2 cup cherry tomatoes, diced
- 1/4 cup red onion, finely chopped
- 1 clove garlic, minced
- 1 tablespoon lime juice
- Salt and pepper to taste
- Fresh cilantro for garnish

Instructions:

1. In a bowl, combine mashed avocados, diced tomatoes, red onion, garlic, lime juice, salt, and pepper.
2. Scoop out a small portion from each cucumber round to create a cup.
3. Fill each cucumber cup with the guacamole mixture.
4. Garnish with fresh cilantro before serving.

Greek Yogurt and Berry Parfait

Ingredients:

- 1 cup Greek yogurt
- 1/2 cup mixed berries (blueberries, strawberries, raspberries)
- 1 tablespoon honey
- 2 tablespoons granola

Instructions:

1. In a glass or bowl, layer Greek yogurt with mixed berries and granola.
2. Drizzle honey over the top.
3. Repeat the layers as desired.

Spicy Roasted Chickpeas

Ingredients:

- 1 can (15 oz) chickpeas, drained and rinsed
- 1 tablespoon olive oil
- 1 teaspoon cumin
- 1/2 teaspoon smoked paprika
- 1/4 teaspoon cayenne pepper
- Salt to taste

Instructions:

1. Preheat the oven to 400°F (200°C).

2. Pat chickpeas dry with a paper towel and toss with olive oil, cumin, smoked paprika, cayenne pepper, and salt.

3. Spread the chickpeas on a baking sheet in a single layer.

4. Roast for 25-30 minutes, shaking the pan halfway through, until chickpeas are crispy.

Caprese Skewers

Ingredients:

- Cherry tomatoes
- Fresh mozzarella balls
- Fresh basil leaves
- Balsamic glaze for drizzling

Instructions:

1. Thread a cherry tomato, a mozzarella ball, and a basil leaf onto small skewers or toothpicks.
2. Arrange the skewers on a serving platter.
3. Drizzle with balsamic glaze before serving.

Apple Slices with Almond Butter

Ingredients:

2 apples, sliced

1/4 cup almond butter

Cinnamon for sprinkling

Instructions:

1. Spread almond butter on apple slices.
2. Sprinkle with cinnamon.
3. Serve immediately for a quick and satisfying snack.

Hummus and Veggie Platter

Ingredients:

- 1 cup hummus
- Assorted veggies (carrot sticks, cucumber slices, cherry tomatoes, bell pepper strips)

Instructions:

1. Arrange the hummus in the center of a platter.
2. Surround the hummus with an assortment of fresh veggies.
3. Dip and enjoy!

Smoked Salmon and Cucumber Bites

Ingredients:

- 1 cucumber, sliced into rounds
- 4 oz smoked salmon

- 2 tablespoons cream cheese
- Fresh dill for garnish

Instructions:

1. Spread a small amount of cream cheese on each cucumber round.
2. Top with a piece of smoked salmon.
3. Garnish with fresh dill before serving.

Berry Smoothie Bowl

Ingredients:

- 1 cup mixed berries (strawberries, blueberries, raspberries)
- 1/2 banana, sliced
- 1/2 cup Greek yogurt
- 1 tablespoon chia seeds
- 2 tablespoons granola

Instructions:

1. Blend mixed berries, banana, and Greek yogurt until smooth.
2. Pour the smoothie into a bowl.
3. Top with chia seeds and granola.

Edamame and Sea Salt Pods

Ingredients:

- 1 cup edamame pods, steamed
- Sea salt to taste

Instructions:

1. Steam edamame pods until tender.
2. Sprinkle with sea salt.
3. Toss to coat and enjoy as a crunchy and nutritious snack.

Baked Sweet Potato Chips

Ingredients:

- 2 sweet potatoes, thinly sliced

- 2 tablespoons olive oil

- 1 teaspoon smoked paprika

- 1/2 teaspoon garlic powder

- Salt to taste

Instructions:

1. Preheat the oven to 400°F (200°C).

2. In a bowl, toss sweet potato slices with olive oil, smoked paprika, garlic powder, and salt.

3. Arrange the slices on a baking sheet in a single layer.

4. Bake for 20-25 minutes or until the chips are crispy.

Avocado and Tomato Salsa

Ingredients:

- 2 avocados, diced

- 1 cup cherry tomatoes, diced
- 1/4 cup red onion, finely chopped
- 1 jalapeño, minced (optional)
- 2 tablespoons lime juice
- Fresh cilantro for garnish
- Salt and pepper to taste

Instructions:

1. In a bowl, combine diced avocados, tomatoes, red onion, jalapeño (if using), lime juice, salt, and pepper.
2. Mix gently to avoid mashing the avocados.
3. Garnish with fresh cilantro before serving.
4. Serve with whole-grain crackers or vegetable slices.

Nut and Seed Trail Mix

Ingredients:

- 1/2 cup almonds
- 1/2 cup walnuts
- 1/4 cup pumpkin seeds
- 1/4 cup sunflower seeds
- 1/4 cup dried cranberries
- 1/4 cup dark chocolate chips

Instructions:

1. In a bowl, mix together almonds, walnuts, pumpkin seeds, sunflower seeds, dried cranberries, and dark chocolate chips.
2. Portion into small snack bags for a convenient on-the-go option.

Cottage Cheese with Pineapple Chunks

Ingredients:

- 1 cup low-fat cottage cheese
- 1 cup pineapple chunks

Instructions:

1. Scoop cottage cheese into a bowl.
2. Top with pineapple chunks.
3. Enjoy this protein-packed and sweet snack.

Stuffed Bell Pepper Halves

Ingredients:

- Bell peppers, halved and seeds removed
- Hummus
- Cherry tomatoes, halved
- Cucumber, diced
- Fresh parsley for garnish

Instructions:

1. Fill each bell pepper half with hummus.

2. Top with cherry tomatoes and diced cucumber.

3. Garnish with fresh parsley before serving.

Rice Cake with Almond Butter and Banana Slices

Ingredients:

- Rice cakes
- Almond butter
- Banana, sliced
- Honey for drizzling

Instructions:

1. Spread almond butter on rice cakes.

2. Top with banana slices.

3. Drizzle with honey for a touch of
   sweetness.

82

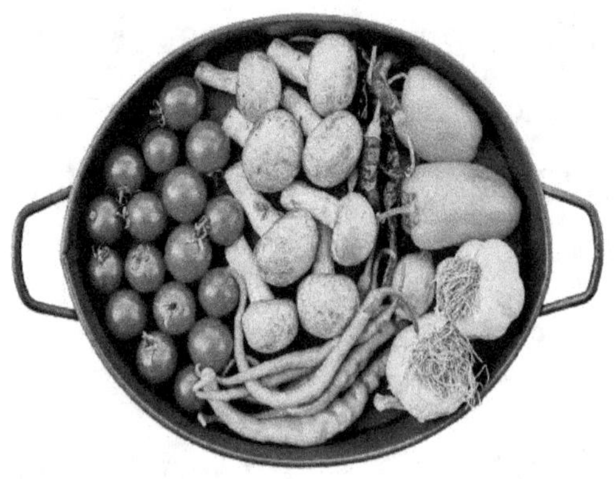

CHAPTER 7: DESSERTS AND TREATS

Chocolate Avocado Mousse

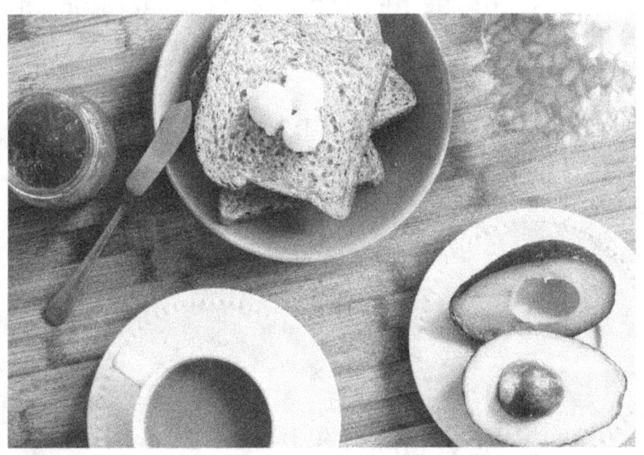

Ingredients:

- 2 ripe avocados
- 1/2 cup unsweetened cocoa powder
- 1/4 cup maple syrup
- 1 teaspoon vanilla extract
- Pinch of salt
- Fresh berries for garnish

Instructions:

1. In a blender, combine avocados, cocoa powder, maple syrup, vanilla extract, and a pinch of salt.
2. Blend until smooth and creamy.
3. Chill the mousse in the refrigerator for at least 30 minutes.
4. Serve topped with fresh berries.

Almond Flour Blueberry Muffins

Ingredients:

- 2 cups almond flour
- 1/2 teaspoon baking soda
- 1/4 teaspoon salt
- 3 eggs
- 1/4 cup coconut oil, melted
- 1/4 cup honey
- 1 teaspoon vanilla extract
- 1 cup fresh or frozen blueberries

Instructions:

1. Preheat the oven to 350°F (175°C) and line a muffin tin with liners.
2. In a bowl, whisk together almond flour, baking soda, and salt.
3. In another bowl, beat eggs, then add melted coconut oil, honey, and vanilla extract.
4. Combine wet and dry ingredients, then fold in blueberries.
5. Divide the batter among muffin cups and bake for 20-25 minutes or until a toothpick comes out clean.

Chia Seed Chocolate Pudding

Ingredients:

- 1/4 cup chia seeds
- 1 cup almond milk

- 2 tablespoons unsweetened cocoa powder
- 2 tablespoons maple syrup
- 1/2 teaspoon vanilla extract
- Sliced strawberries for garnish

Instructions:

1. In a jar, combine chia seeds, almond milk, cocoa powder, maple syrup, and vanilla extract.
2. Stir well, cover, and refrigerate for at least 2 hours or overnight.
3. Stir again before serving and top with sliced strawberries.

Coconut Flour Banana Bread

Ingredients:

- 1/2 cup coconut flour
- 1/2 teaspoon baking soda

- 1/4 teaspoon salt
- 3 ripe bananas, mashed
- 3 eggs
- 1/4 cup coconut oil, melted
- 1 teaspoon vanilla extract
- 1/2 cup chopped walnuts (optional)

Instructions:

1. Preheat the oven to 350°F (175°C) and grease a loaf pan.
2. In a bowl, mix coconut flour, baking soda, and salt.
3. In another bowl, combine mashed bananas, eggs, melted coconut oil, and vanilla extract.
4. Add the wet ingredients to the dry ingredients and mix until well combined.
5. Fold in chopped walnuts if desired.
6. Pour the batter into the prepared loaf pan and bake for 40-45 minutes or until a toothpick comes out clean.

Berry and Almond Flour Crisp

Ingredients:

- 2 cups mixed berries (strawberries, blueberries, raspberries)
- 1 tablespoon arrowroot powder
- 1 tablespoon lemon juice
- 1 cup almond flour
- 1/4 cup coconut oil, melted
- 1/4 cup maple syrup
- 1/2 cup sliced almonds

Instructions:

1. Preheat the oven to 350°F (175°C) and grease a baking dish.
2. In a bowl, toss mixed berries with arrowroot powder and lemon juice, then spread them in the baking dish.

3. In another bowl, mix almond flour, melted coconut oil, and maple syrup.

4. Sprinkle the almond flour mixture over the berries and top with sliced almonds.

5. Bake for 25-30 minutes or until the topping is golden brown.

Avocado Chocolate Chip Cookies

Ingredients:

- 2 ripe avocados, mashed
- 1/2 cup coconut sugar
- 1 egg
- 1 teaspoon vanilla extract
- 2 cups almond flour
- 1/2 teaspoon baking soda
- 1/4 teaspoon salt
- 1/2 cup dark chocolate chips

Instructions:

1. Preheat the oven to 350°F (175°C) and line a baking sheet with parchment paper.
2. In a bowl, cream together mashed avocados, coconut sugar, egg, and vanilla extract.
3. In another bowl, whisk together almond flour, baking soda, and salt.
4. Combine wet and dry ingredients, then fold in dark chocolate chips.
5. Drop spoonfuls of dough onto the baking sheet and bake for 10-12 minutes or until the edges are golden.

Greek Yogurt Parfait with Honey and Berries

Ingredients:

- 1 cup Greek yogurt
- 2 tablespoons honey

- 1/2 cup granola
- 1 cup mixed berries (strawberries, blueberries, raspberries)

Instructions:

- In a glass or bowl, layer Greek yogurt with honey, granola, and mixed berries.
- Repeat the layers as desired.
- Drizzle with additional honey before serving.

Pumpkin Spice Chia Pudding

Ingredients:

- 1/4 cup chia seeds
- 1 cup almond milk
- 1/4 cup canned pumpkin
- 2 tablespoons maple syrup
- 1/2 teaspoon pumpkin spice
- Whipped coconut cream for garnish

Instructions:

1. In a jar, combine chia seeds, almond milk, canned pumpkin, maple syrup, and pumpkin spice.
2. Stir well, cover, and refrigerate for at least 2 hours or overnight.
3. Top with whipped coconut cream before serving.

Almond Butter Energy Bites

Ingredients:

- 1 cup rolled oats
- 1/2 cup almond butter
- 1/4 cup honey
- 1/4 cup dark chocolate chips
- 1/4 cup shredded coconut
- 1 teaspoon vanilla extract
- Pinch of salt

Instructions:

1. In a bowl, mix together rolled oats, almond butter, honey, dark chocolate chips, shredded coconut, vanilla extract, and a pinch of salt.

2. Form the mixture into bite-sized balls and refrigerate for at least 30 minutes before serving.

Coconut Lime Energy Balls

Ingredients:

- 1 cup shredded coconut
- 1/2 cup cashews
- 1/4 cup coconut oil, melted
- Zest and juice of 1 lime
- 2 tablespoons honey
- 1 teaspoon vanilla extract
- Pinch of salt

Instructions:

1. In a food processor, blend shredded coconut and cashews until finely ground.

2. Add melted coconut oil, lime zest, lime juice, honey, vanilla extract, and a pinch of salt. Blend until well combined.

3. Roll the mixture into small balls and refrigerate for at least 30 minutes before serving.

Chocolate Covered Strawberries

Ingredients:

- 1 cup dark chocolate chips
- 1 pound strawberries, washed and dried

Instructions:

1. Melt dark chocolate chips in a microwave-safe bowl, stirring every 30 seconds until smooth.

2. Dip each strawberry into the melted chocolate, allowing excess to drip off.

3. Place the dipped strawberries on a parchment-lined tray and refrigerate until the chocolate hardens.

Cinnamon Baked Apples

Ingredients:

- 4 apples, cored and halved
- 2 tablespoons melted coconut oil
- 2 teaspoons ground cinnamon
- 1 tablespoon honey
- Chopped nuts for garnish (optional)

Instructions:

1. Preheat the oven to 375°F (190°C).

2. In a bowl, toss apple halves with melted coconut oil and ground cinnamon.
3. Place the apples on a baking sheet, drizzle with honey, and bake for 20-25 minutes or until tender.
4. Garnish with chopped nuts if desired.

Mixed Berry Sorbet

Ingredients:

- 2 cups mixed berries (strawberries, blueberries, raspberries)
- 1/4 cup honey
- 1 tablespoon lemon juice

Instructions:

1. In a blender, combine mixed berries, honey, and lemon juice.
2. Blend until smooth.

3. Pour the mixture into a shallow dish and freeze for at least 4 hours, stirring every hour.

4. Scoop the sorbet into bowls and serve.

Lemon Poppy Seed Muffins

Ingredients:

- 2 cups almond flour
- 1/2 teaspoon baking soda
- 1/4 teaspoon salt
- Zest and juice of 2 lemons
- 3 eggs
- 1/4 cup coconut oil, melted
- 1/4 cup honey
- 1 teaspoon vanilla extract
- 1 tablespoon poppy seeds

Instructions:

1. Preheat the oven to 350°F (175°C) and line a muffin tin with liners.
2. In a bowl, whisk together almond flour, baking soda, and salt.
3. In another bowl, mix lemon zest, lemon juice, eggs, melted coconut oil, honey, and vanilla extract.
4. Combine wet and dry ingredients, then fold in poppy seeds.
5. Divide the batter among muffin cups and bake for 20-25 minutes or until a toothpick comes out clean.

Raspberry Coconut Chia Popsicles

Ingredients:

- 1 cup coconut milk
- 1 cup raspberries
- 2 tablespoons chia seeds
- 1 tablespoon honey

Instructions:

1. In a blender, combine coconut milk, raspberries, chia seeds, and honey.

2. Blend until smooth.

3. Pour the mixture into popsicle molds and freeze for at least 4 hours before serving

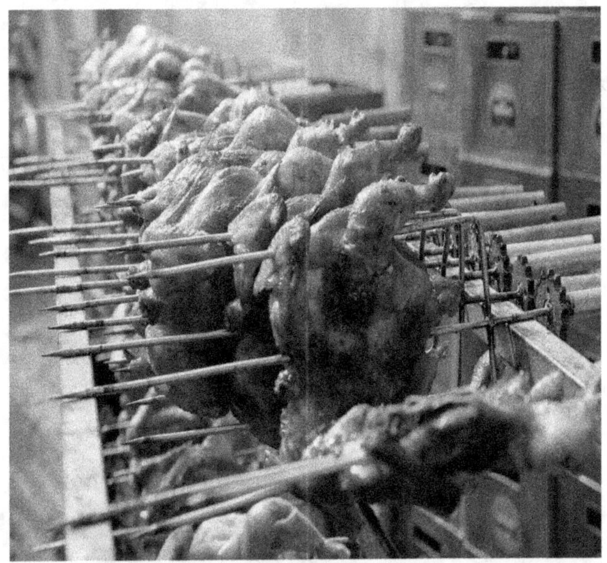

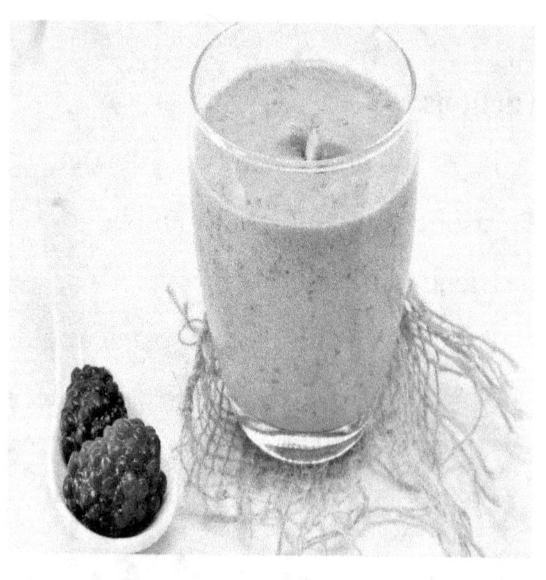

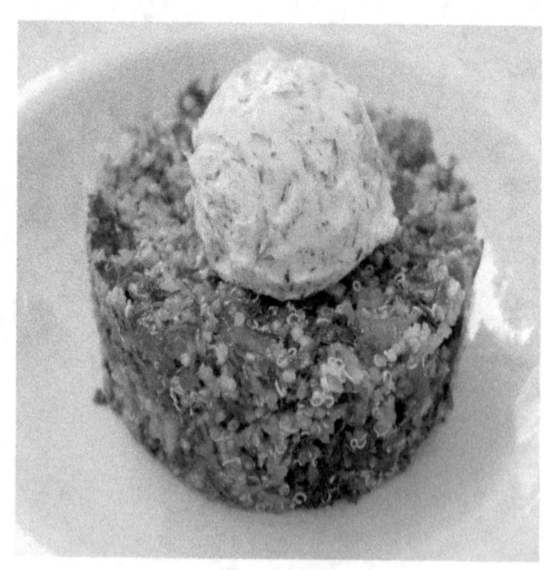

CHAPTER 8: SMOOTHIE AND BEVERAGES RECIPES

Green Detox Smoothie

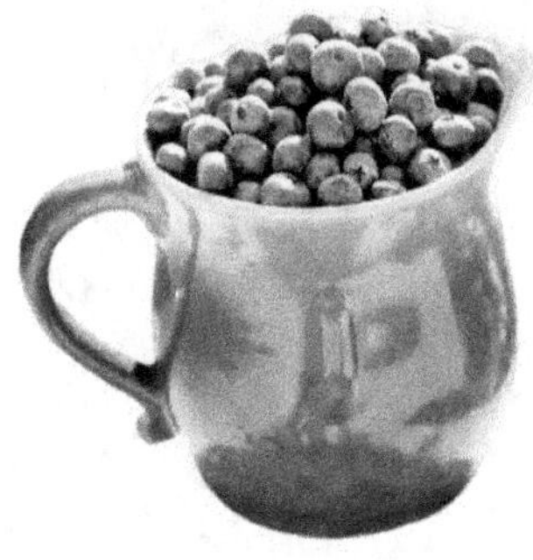

Ingredients:

- 1 cup kale, stems removed
- 1/2 cucumber, peeled and sliced
- 1/2 green apple, cored and chopped
- 1/2 lemon, juiced
- 1 tablespoon chia seeds

- 1 cup coconut water
- Ice cubes (optional)

Instructions:

1. In a blender, combine kale, cucumber, green apple, lemon juice, chia seeds, and coconut water.
2. Blend until smooth.
3. Add ice cubes if desired and blend again.
4. Pour into a glass and enjoy the refreshing detox smoothie.

Berry Protein Smoothie

Ingredients:

- 1 cup mixed berries (strawberries, blueberries, raspberries)
- 1/2 banana
- 1 scoop vanilla protein powder
- 1 tablespoon almond butter

- 1 cup almond milk
- Ice cubes (optional)

Instructions:

1. Blend mixed berries, banana, vanilla protein powder, almond butter, and almond milk until smooth.
2. Add ice cubes if a colder consistency is preferred.
3. Pour into a glass and savor the protein-packed berry goodness.

Tropical Turmeric Smoothie

Ingredients:
- 1/2 cup pineapple chunks
- 1/2 mango, peeled and diced
- 1/2 teaspoon turmeric powder
- 1 tablespoon chia seeds
- 1 cup coconut water

- Ice cubes (optional)

Instructions:

1. Blend pineapple, mango, turmeric powder, chia seeds, and coconut water until smooth.
2. Add ice cubes if desired and blend again.
3. Pour into a glass for a tropical turmeric delight.

Cucumber Mint Cooler

Ingredients:

- 1 cucumber, peeled and sliced
- 1/4 cup fresh mint leaves
- 1 lime, juiced
- 1 tablespoon honey
- 2 cups water
- Ice cubes

Instructions:

1. In a blender, combine cucumber slices, mint leaves, lime juice, honey, and water.
2. Blend until well combined.
3. Strain the mixture to remove pulp if desired.
4. Serve over ice for a refreshing cucumber mint cooler.

Golden Milk Latte

Ingredients:

1. 1 cup unsweetened almond milk
2. 1/2 teaspoon turmeric powder
3. 1/4 teaspoon cinnamon
4. Pinch of black pepper
5. 1 teaspoon honey or maple syrup (optional)

Instructions:

1. In a small saucepan, heat almond milk over medium heat.

2. Whisk in turmeric, cinnamon, black pepper, and honey or maple syrup.

3. Heat until the mixture is warmed through but not boiling.

4. Pour into a mug and enjoy the comforting golden milk latte.

Blueberry Avocado Smoothie

Ingredients:

- 1/2 avocado
- 1 cup blueberries
- 1/2 banana
- 1 cup coconut water
- 1 tablespoon flaxseeds
- Ice cubes (optional)

Instructions:

1. Blend avocado, blueberries, banana, coconut water, and flaxseeds until smooth.

2. Add ice cubes if desired and blend again.

3. Pour into a glass for a creamy and nutritious blueberry avocado smoothie.

Minty Watermelon Refresher

Ingredients:

- 2 cups watermelon, cubed
- 1/4 cup fresh mint leaves
- 1 lime, juiced
- 1 tablespoon honey
- 2 cups water
- Ice cubes

Instructions:

1. In a blender, combine watermelon, mint leaves, lime juice, honey, and water.

2. Blend until smooth.

3. Strain the mixture to remove pulp if desired.

4. Serve over ice for a cooling and hydrating watermelon refresher.

Chocolate Peanut Butter Protein Shake

Ingredients:

- 1 cup unsweetened almond milk
- 1 scoop chocolate protein powder
- 1 tablespoon peanut butter
- 1/2 banana
- Ice cubes (optional)

Instructions:

1. Blend almond milk, chocolate protein powder, peanut butter, and banana until smooth.

2. Add ice cubes if desired and blend again.

3. Pour into a glass for a delicious chocolate peanut butter protein shake.

Pineapple Ginger Turmeric Elixir

Ingredients:

- 1 cup pineapple chunks
- 1-inch piece of ginger, peeled
- 1/2 teaspoon turmeric powder
- 1 tablespoon honey
- 2 cups water
- Ice cubes

Instructions:

1. In a blender, combine pineapple chunks, ginger, turmeric powder, honey, and water.

2. Blend until well combined.

3. Strain the mixture to remove pulp if desired.

4. Serve over ice for a zesty and immune-boosting elixir.

Vanilla Almond Chai Smoothie

Ingredients:

- 1 cup unsweetened almond milk
- 1/2 teaspoon vanilla extract
- 1 chai tea bag, steeped and cooled
- 1 scoop vanilla protein powder
- 1 tablespoon almond butter
- Ice cubes (optional)

Instructions:

1. In a blender, combine almond milk, vanilla extract, cooled chai tea, vanilla protein powder, and almond butter.

2. Add ice cubes if desired and blend until smooth.

3. Pour into a glass for a comforting vanilla almond chai smoothie

Raspberry Coconut Water Refresher

Ingredients:

- 1 cup raspberries
- 1/2 cup coconut water
- 1 tablespoon chia seeds
- 1 teaspoon honey
- 1 cup water
- Ice cubes

Instructions:

1. Blend raspberries, coconut water, chia seeds, honey, and water until smooth.

2. Strain the mixture to remove seeds if desired.

3. Serve over ice for a hydrating and antioxidant-rich refresher.

Matcha Green Tea Latte

Ingredients:

- 1 teaspoon matcha powder
- 1 cup unsweetened almond milk
- 1 teaspoon honey or maple syrup (optional)

Instructions:

1. In a small bowl, whisk matcha powder with a small amount of almond milk to form a paste.

2. Heat the remaining almond milk in a saucepan until warmed but not boiling.

3. Whisk the matcha paste into the warmed almond milk until well combined.

4. Sweeten with honey or maple syrup if desired.

5. Pour into a mug and enjoy the energizing matcha green tea latte.

Orange Creamsicle Smoothie

Ingredients:

- 1 cup orange segments
- 1/2 banana
- 1/2 cup Greek yogurt
- 1/2 teaspoon vanilla extract
- 1 tablespoon chia seeds
- Ice cubes (optional)

Instructions:

1. Blend orange segments, banana, Greek yogurt, vanilla extract, and chia seeds until smooth.

2. Add ice cubes if desired and blend again.

3. Pour into a glass for a citrusy and creamy orange creamsicle smoothie.

Peach Mint Iced Tea

Ingredients:

- 2 peaches, sliced
- 1/4 cup fresh mint leaves
- 2 black tea bags
- 1 tablespoon honey
- 4 cups water
- Ice cubes

Instructions:

1. In a saucepan, bring water to a boil and steep the black tea bags.

2. Add sliced peaches, mint leaves, and honey to the hot tea.

3. Allow the mixture to cool, then refrigerate until cold.

4. Serve over ice for a refreshing peach mint iced tea.

Coconut Berry Smoothie Bowl

Ingredients:

- 1/2 cup mixed berries (strawberries, blueberries, raspberries)
- 1/2 banana
- 1/2 cup coconut milk
- 1 tablespoon unsweetened shredded coconut
- Toppings: sliced almonds, chia seeds, fresh berries

Instructions:

1. Blend mixed berries, banana, coconut milk, and shredded coconut until smooth.
2. Pour the smoothie into a bowl.
3. Top with sliced almonds, chia seeds, and fresh berries for a delightful coconut berry smoothie bowl.

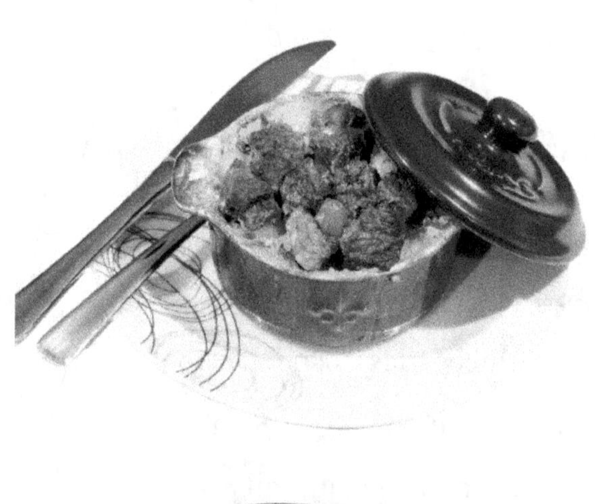

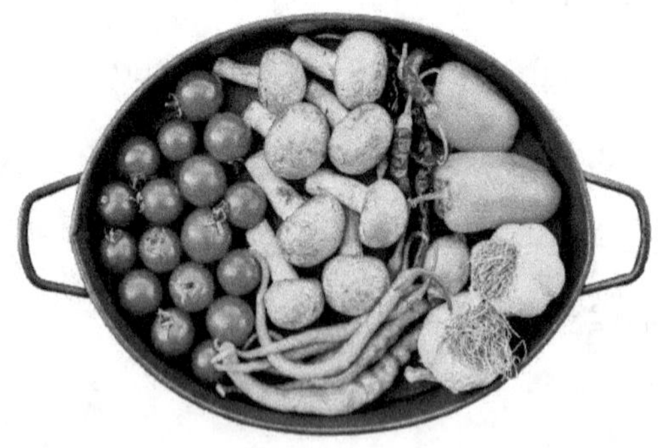

CONCLUSION

ADDITIONAL RESOURCES

In conclusion, the Galveston Diet Cookbook stands not only as a collection of recipes but as a guiding light on the path to holistic well-being. It embodies a philosophy that transcends conventional diets, offering a lifestyle centered around nourishment, balance, and mindfulness. For individuals like Paul, it becomes a transformative tool, unlocking the secrets to vitality and providing a tangible, flavorful roadmap to a healthier existence.

As the pages of the cookbook unfold, so does a narrative of resilience and triumph over health challenges. It empowers individuals to reclaim control over their health, fostering a positive relationship with food that extends beyond mere sustenance. The cookbook encapsulates the essence of a community bound by a common goal — the pursuit of optimal health in the coastal charm of Galveston.

Complementary resources, such as the community forum, blog, app, and wellness coaching, enrich the Galveston Diet experience. They provide a supportive ecosystem for individuals to share experiences, gain knowledge, and receive personalized guidance, ensuring that the journey to well-being is not a solitary one.

In the realm of the Galveston Diet, individuals discover not just a culinary guide but a holistic approach to life. It's a journey marked by flavorful recipes, mindful choices, and a newfound appreciation for the profound impact of nutrition on overall health. The Galveston Diet Cookbook, along with its supplementary resources, serves as an invaluable companion, inspiring individuals to embrace a vibrant and revitalized lifestyle in the coastal haven of Galveston.

www.ingramcontent.com/pod-product-compliance
Lightning Source LLC
Chambersburg PA
CBHW070856260726
48661CB00004B/1441